Why and how

SURYA NAMASKAR?

Easy – Effective - YOGA Practice

Ayem

Kindle Direct Publishing

Dedicated to wonderful teacher

Ms Jyotsna Narayanan

Contents

Acknowledgements

I thank Krishnamacharya Yoga Mandiram, Vinieyoga Healing Centre, Shamkaram, Yogavahini, Tamil Nadu Sports University and Ashtanga Vinyasa Yoga for the opportunity to learn yoga in general and Surya Namaskar in particular.

I am grateful to all my teachers in general and Sri Lara Abiesheik, Ms Srimathi and Sri Srivatsa Ramaswami who have helped me to know more about Surya Namaskar (SN).

I thank the yoga fraternity, my friends and co-teachers.

I thank Ms Sandhya Sundar who has corrected and edited the text passionately. Her knowledge of yoga, philosophy and of course expertise in language has been very helpful to make the book better.

I especially thank Mr O S Rajendran for his asana stick drawings, Ms Sumathi Vinayagamoorthi for her feedback and minute corrections, Mr C Arumugam for the interior design, Ms Sathya Ganapathy for the wrapper image and Mr Vijay Amarnath for the wrapper design.

Yoga students and yoga teachers who have participated in my yoga classes and who have shared their experiences with me also gave me an opportunity to learn from them. I thank all of them.

This book has become possible because of the help I have received from all of you. I thank everyone who made this effort possible.

I look forward to working with all of you again.

Preface

"Surya Namaskar is an all-round practice for all, young and old, men and women. The truth is as real and as clear as the sun in the sky. It requires no canvassing to prove its worth. It is a real training to our body soul and mind."

Subhash Bhagwantrao Khardekar

'suryanamaskar.info'.

Life gives us opportunities to do wonders, but how many of us are able to use these opportunities effectively? We struggle even to do our routine work and so we complain, blame, find fault ... one of the main reasons for our struggle is poor health.

We think about doing so many activities but our body doesn't cooperate with us. So, we compromise, postpone and cancel. In this process we are disturbed a lot. Procrastination becomes our nature, so that even in the planning stage we shrink our ideas and start thinking small. Reason: poor health!

We have time for entertainment, gadgets, making calls, visiting places, anything except exercising. Even if we decide to exercise, we are not able to execute it. It remains in the mind. Some of us start, but dropout soon. **Only a very few decide, plan well, execute effectively and enjoy good health and life**.

My friend Raju has been thinking about doing something for his health, but has not been able to do so for many months. Nothing materializes for him; he is not sure what to do; he does not have clarity; he is fearful of doing something new and doubts the benefits of any practice. There are many health practices but which is the one that will take care of his whole system in a short time?

Me: Hello Raju, what are your thoughts about exercise? Have you decided anything?

Raju: Hello, no, I still have questions. I am not sure what the right health regimen is for me.

Me: There are so many, from walking to yoga. What do you want to do?

Raju: I am always busy so can't spare much time. I need something short and easy.

Me: Why do you want to exercise, Raju?

Raju: To be fit, not to have disease, to be young, to be more active, to sleep well, to reduce weight, to have good digestion, to have more energy … it is a big list.

Me: Oh interesting. You want so many benefits but are not ready to spend time.

Raju: Not exactly. I can somehow spare 30 minutes maximum.

Me: What about regular walking?

Raju: Not interested. I feel tired after a walk. Besides, I have to buy shoes, find the right place to walk, get up early. I have to prepare for that, sorry.

Me: What about going to the gym?

Raju: I have to go to the gym, pay fees, buy shoes and other accessories. It is very difficult. So suggest something short and easy to do without fancy equipment and expenditure.

Me: Then why don't you think about Surya Namaskar (SN) practice?

Raju: Sorry I can't get up early in the morning and also, I have heard that it is difficult to do.

Me: If not in the early morning, you can practice SN when you get up. In 24 hours can't you find 20 to 30 minutes (mins) for your health?

Me: Raju: Will 20 to 30 mins be enough? Then I will try.

Me: In my experience, the busiest people also somehow find time for a health regimen and they practice every day. They understand that health is very important. So they make every day count.

Raju: Ok ok. I will consider. Tell me something about SN now.

Me: SN is an ancient system comprising 12 postures and it has been practiced for thousands of years. It is very powerful and has proven to be highly beneficial. Are you really interested?

Raju: Yes, very much.

Me: Here are some points for you to think about:

- SN has been designed excellently.
- It doesn't take much time.
- SN takes care of the whole human system.
- The benefits are many.
- It has many variations.
- You can choose to do as many rounds as you want, according to your need, time and ability.
- It will help you focus on your activities far better.

In the world of SN there are many practices: As a ritual, with mantra, with namaskars, in the morning, 108 times, during sun rise … all demand discipline.

You can practice SN at any time. It is also easy, effective and can be practiced anywhere. Our ancestors didn't know you and your busy schedule but they have created SN to suit our hectic life style.

Raju: What is the proof that SN works well and is beneficial?

Me: I have been practicing it for the past 30 years. As a yoga teacher, I have been teaching and have seen how SN brings great changes and impacts practitioners. It makes the practitioners healthier and happier. Most importantly, it is suitable for people like you.

The 12 steps of SN have made changes in millions of people across nations. There is so much to explore.

Raju: Go on, my dear friend.

Me: I have written this book for people like you. It is a guide to practice SN. However, if you have any health issues do consult a general physician or an Ayurvedic Vaidya or a yoga therapist who has special training in handling health issues before you begin the practice.

Raju: It's very interesting; I will try SN soon.

All the very best Raju!

P.S. This book follows Sri Krishnamacharya's school of yoga. **Tirumalai Krishnamacharya** (November 18, 1888 – February 28, 1989) was an Ayurvedic healer and scholar. He taught classical asana, yoga therapy, yoga philosophy and also Vedic chanting. He is often referred to as 'the father of modern yoga'.

Krishnamacharya Yoga Mandiram (KYM) was started to spread his teaching and I am fortunate to have studied in his yoga school. I teach asanas and pranayama primarily to groups.

Ayem
ayemyoga@gmail.com

Chapter 1

Yoga Power

"Yoga is an intimately personal and deeply experiential. Only the practitioner experiences yoga. In fact, yoga is a manifestation of the total inner potential of every individual."

Dr. N. Chandrasekaran
Principles and Practice of Yoga Therapy – Book 1.

Yoga is a system which is very powerful and is capable of making us transform from fit to great. Today this is one of the fastest growing practices across the world. It is very dear to millions of people. It grows with technology and media too – so it has been reaching all parts of the globe and makes positive changes in human lives.

Why does the whole world practice yoga? Is it because it is so popular? Or because is it an ancient Indian system? Or it has great varieties and choices? Or is it because one can practice it anywhere at any time? I believe that it must be due to its impact on the practitioners and the way it changes their lives. **So they like it, love it, adore it, many see it as a source of great health, happiness and peace. Hence, they make Yoga a part of their lives!**

Every day so many yoga events happen across the globe. Starting from launching new yoga centres – studios, organising seminars, retreats, yoga training programs, satsangs, yoga shops to marathons connected to yoga, publications, videos, online classes, and lectures, and also celebration of the International Day of Yoga.

After practice, yoga practitioners share their experiences through their writing, videos and training. They are able to reach many people online. To address the people's need for yoga, many become yoga teachers and trainers. In this connection Indian yoga teachers and therapists go abroad and many yoga lovers, teachers from abroad come to India to learn the system in its birth place.

Today the yoga fraternity has become a beautiful world and tens of thousands of practitioners live through yoga teachings and other yoga related activities. So where there is a business, income and job opportunities, there yoga naturally expands its horizons.

In yoga, besides the traditional yoga practices of different yoga schools, there are many types of modern yoga practices. Many are eager to know the new ones and yoga studios are promoting such practices.

A few examples for modern yoga types:

Aerial Yoga: Using a hammock-like strap to hang from the ceiling and practicing asanas off the floor.

Laughter Yoga: Laughter Yoga allows us to get together in a group and just laugh. The fake laugh eventually turns into a real laugh.

Chair yoga: It is primarily meant for elderly people and also who have challenges in doing normal asana practice.

BROGA: This type is invented by men, for men. It focuses around strength training, muscle toning and cardiovascular work.

SUP Yoga: Practicing yoga on a stand-up paddleboard.

Yoga HIIT: This is a great option for those who want a quick, high-tempo take on yoga.

Chromayog: A practise which uses colour, light and music to create a multi-sensory experience. Chroma Yoga is also known as Light Therapy Yoga.

Goat Yoga: Practicing yoga amidst goats.

There is also, **Snake yoga, Eco yoga, Acro yoga, Doga, Naked yoga, Beer yoga** and so on.

In this expansive trend, yoga has also entered almost all the fields from sports, medicine, performing arts, corporate businesses, education ... It plays a role and impact wherever it is used effectively.

The beauty of yoga is that children, students, youngsters, married people, aged people ... all ages and all genders have space to practice and get benefits from it and make life better, more beautiful. Yoga is such a vast system and creates space for anyone who approaches it in an appropriate way.

Besides, **Yoga Therapy** is become popular today in many countries. It is addressing health issues and brings positive changes in thousands of people. Here yoga experts and yoga therapists use yoga tools and modify according to the ill persons' need and level to design a practice that will give the required benefits. 'The International Association of Yoga Therapists (IAYT) represents more than 5,600 yoga and healthcare professionals working in more than 50 countries. The organization supports research and education in yoga as therapy and serves as a professional resource for yoga therapists and yoga teachers.' https://yogatherapy.health/about-iayt/

Even though yoga is popular in every country, that doesn't mean all people know about it well and they practice it regularly. But **the one who practices yoga properly at the right time and in the right way enjoys its benefits and experiences exclusively.**

If the demands of yoga practice are fulfilled, there won't be a shortage of benefits and rare changes. Many feel that yoga is a great practice for experiences and for inner peace.

So, **yoga does open its doors to those who are sincere, consistent, have faith and look forward to the system with eagerness. They are able to see things in a new light.**

How does yoga work?

Yoga is a practice which is ancient and also modern. So, one has to understand the nuances, techniques, traditions, importance and practical details of yoga well before starting to practice it.

Yoga works at the following five levels.

- Annamaya kosa - physical level

- Pranamaya kosa - energy level

- Manomaya kosa - mind level

- Vignanamaya kosa - personality level

- Anandamaya kosa– great joy level

Many texts discuss the functions, effects and benefits of yoga in detail. Because of its extraordinary power, layers of depth and vast space for anyone from the ordinary to one who has experienced the highest, it is capable of taking care of the world in a healthy way!

Note however that while most people label their practice as yoga, more than 80% of them do only asanas. Benefits occur in accordance with the quality and regularity of appropriate practice. There are many approaches and styles in asana practice. Some start with simple asanas, some start with more intense asanas, some classes introduce more stretches, while others bring in bandhas (internal holds).

Apart from this, some repeat the same set of asanas during practice, while others may keep introducing new asanas now and then. Practice could be slow and involve deep breathing or it could be with counts for breathing. Some practitioners enjoy standing asanas, some enjoy inverted asanas like sirshasana, sarvangasana, halasana and so on, while many more enjoy sitting and lying postures. Even in standing asanas, some choose to practise twists, some favour back arches or forward bends. Hundreds of practices are possible!

However, **yoga does not mean only asana practice and physical fitness. Deeper experiences, greater results and transformations are possible.** For such an experience, however, one needs commitment, great effort and regular practice for a very long period of time.

If practitioners include pranayama along with asanas, they will be able to regulate their breathing – which means making the breath long, subtle and deep, and holding the breath inside or out. Some may prefer to spend more time doing asanas, while aged people may prefer pranayama. From flexibility to a quiet mind many benefits are achievable through dedicated practice.

Also, if practitioners could add the first two steps of Patanjali's Ashtanga yoga (which means the eight components of yoga) – yama and niyama (discipline in the outer world and within oneself) to asana and pranayama, then the whole practice will reach more sublime levels. Not only will the practice be deeper and better; a marked improvement will be seen in one's nature, approach, activities, thoughts and feelings. "These eight steps basically act as guidelines on how to live a meaningful and purposeful life. They serve as a prescription for moral and ethical conduct and self-discipline; they direct attention toward one's health, and they help us to acknowledge the spiritual aspects of our nature." -https://www.yogajournal.com/practice/the-eight-limbs.

What is important in yoga practice is that one finds the right yoga tradition and the right yoga teacher for suitable guidance.

I am fortunate to see people changing a lot through yoga practice; they calm their mind and focus it in a productive direction. Yoga practices are also very effective in addressing mind distractions, attention deficiency, stress, sleep disorders, digestion-related issues, and so on.

As many experienced yogis say, yoga is an ocean. We can see it, we can go into it, we can swim in it, we can travel in it, we can make it a part of us ... the possibilities are many. How we see yoga, how we relate to it, how we deal with it and how long we stay with it will determine the benefits and experiences.

The beauty of yoga is that with the right guidance, anybody can start practicing at any age, at any level of fitness. Those who practice it regularly, making a lifelong commitment to it, will understand the various levels, choices, depths, layers, many details, and the many nuances of yoga. In that yoga journey, they will experience its power and its ability to transform.

Chapter 2

Surya Namaskar: An Introduction

'Surya Namaskar awakens the solar aspects of an individual's nature and releases this vital energy for the development of higher awareness. This [awareness] can be realized by the practice of Surya Namaskar each morning. [The practice is also] a fine way to pay tribute to the source of creation and life, [allowing us] thereby [to] carry on the solar tradition.'

Swamy Satyananda Saraswati
Surya Namaskara: A Technique of Solar Vitalization

Surya Namaskar (Surya means Sun, namaskar means salutation = Sun Salutation) is one of the early ritual practices of India. People used the form to respect the Sun God. SN was practiced daily in the morning during sunrise and it has been transferred from generation to generation. Now it is very popular across the globe.

'The Sun is the divine source of energy and has been worshipped around the world. The Greeks called the Sun god Helius; the Romans referred to him as Titan and Hyperoin; the Egyptians called him Ra. In Mexican culture, he is Kikich Ahau; the Germans call the sun Sol; in Chinese culture, the sun represents Yang (Pingala) and the Moon represents Yin (Ida).'- *fractalenlightenment.com*/14413/spirituality/surya-namaskar

The ancient way of doing Sun Salutation in India was to chant mantras during the practice and to prostrate to the sun god by placing the whole body on the earth and stretching the arms in front. The whole sequence was repeated a number of times in the mornings.

Another form of SN was practiced inside homes. Expert practitioners of SN were invited to homes to perform it 108 times accompanied by mantras. In some families, members too joined the practice. But many used to only watch the practice and listen to the mantras.

Subramaniya Sastrikal, an SN practitioner, used to practice SN in two to three houses in a morning. He shared his SN experiences with a colleague and me in 2014:

"Specifically, they used to watch me, whether I am doing the SN properly with the mantra. In the month of December, I used to have more opportunities to do the Namaskar in many houses. Because of SN practice in my young age, now in my 103rd year, I am able to manage myself well and have no diabetes or blood pressure."

Both forms were practiced for hundreds of years in India. In fact, there were many more rituals to pay respect to the Sun God. However, whether inside the home or outside, the practices were performed with mantras, in the morning time.

These practices of SN have undergone so many changes that what the majority of people practice today is mostly without mantras and without the sun too!

In SN, there are 12 steps and each step focuses on one area of our body. Every step has a breath component. SN pulls the muscles of the whole body, activates the joints and moves all parts of the body. Each step is a precursor to the next.

Those who have practiced SN will probably understand my next statements. When one has completed a few rounds of SN, the body feels light, stretched and energized. These sensations can be physically felt both inside the body and externally. This can be felt even within a few minutes of practice.

There is much depth, nuance, perfection and intelligence in the way SN has been put together. Wise practitioners today will

remain with it and gather the extraordinary health benefits that happen naturally, whether they specifically look forward to it or not.

Mantras are commonly used in SN practice. The most common mantras are listed below. Mantra worship of the sun is common in India.

> Recitation of the Veda-s has several benefits when practiced in the right manner. The Veda-s are the source of most of the mantra-s that are in practice. **The mantra-s are powerful sounds, which when pronounced in the right manner produce certain vibrations that have the potential to alter our physiological state, thereby improving physical and mental health.** This is why mantra-s have been used for many years in India as a means of personal and spiritual transformation … and **another benefit of Vedic chanting is the ability to bring the mind to a state of complete attention.**
>
> **TKV Desikachar**
> *Mantra Mala*

The following mantra is a verbal salutation to the sun. It has been taken from the *Taittiriya Upanishad*

uddyannadya mitramahaḥ

ārohannuttarām divam

hrdrogam mama sūrya

harimāṇam ca nāśaya

śukeṣu me harimāṇam

ropaṇākāsu dadhmasi

atho hāridraveṣu me

harimāṇam nidadhmasi|

udagādayamādityaḥ

viṣvena sahasā saha

dviṣantam mama randhayan

mo aham dviṣato ratham

All living beings of this divine creation depend on the Sun as it removes physical, mental and spiritual weakness. The seven colours of the Sun are very important for a person and chanting the Surya Mantra will help absorb the positivity of these colours. Also, early morning bathing followed with sun bathing, while offering your gratitude and respect to Surya Deva [while] chanting the Surya mantra is so beneficial for your body [that] one can heal their body of all ailments and increase intelligence.

https://www.speakingtree.in/blog/surya-mantra

In Surya Namaskar practice, we have two types of mantras: bija mantras and SN mantras.

I. Surya Namaskar -Bija Mantras

- **Om hiram**

- **Om hrim**

- **Om hrum**

- **Om hroum**

- **Om hrim**

- **Om hraha**

II. Surya Namaskar Mantras

S.No. Mantra	Meaning
1. **Om mitrāya namaḥ**	Salutations to the one who is friendly to all.
2. **Om ravaye namaḥ**	Salutations to the one who is the cause for change.
3. **Om suryāya namaḥ**	Salutations to the one who induces activity .
4. **Om bhānave namaḥ**	Salutations to the one who diffuses Light
5. **Om khagāya namaḥ**	Salutations to the one who moves through the sky.
6. **Om pūṣaṇe namaḥ**	Salutations to the one who gives nourishment and fulfillment.
7. **Om hiraṇyagarbhāya namaḥ**	Salutations to the one who contains everything.
8. **Om maricāyanamaḥ**	Salutations to the one who possesses rays.
9. **Om ādityāyanamaḥ**	Salutations to the one who is the son of Aditi
10. **Om savitrenamaḥ**	Salutations to the one who produces everything
11. **Om arkāyanamaḥ**	Salutations to the one who is fit to be worshipped.
12. **Om bhāskarāyanamaḥ**	Salutations to the one who illumines the external and the internal world.

The benefits of SN as it is being practiced currently has been experienced by many scholars and yoga experts, and they have expressed it well in inspiring words:

The SN sequence not only wakes up the body but also "calls us to stretch our minds and spirits to the corners of the universe, allowing us to feel the vast expanse of the cosmos within the movement of our bodies. As we sweep our arms up and bow forward, we honor the earth, the heavens, and all of life in between that is nourished by the breath cycle. As we lower our bodies, we connect with the earth. As we rise up from the earth, we stretch through the atmosphere once more, reaching for the sky. As we bring our hands together in Namaste, we gather the space of the heavens back into our heart and breath, acknowledging that our body forms the center point between heaven and earth.

Prof. Christopher Key Chapple
https://www.yogajournal.com/yoga-101/shine/

Sun Salutation is considered so profound that many people practice it. It works well for people of all ages, from children to seniors. Respected for its excellent effects, the sun salutation reputedly provides an array of physical benefits, such as stretching the spine and strengthening the muscles that support it; improving posture, coordination, and endurance; and improving lung function and oxygen delivery to cells. Yoga masters claim that the sun salutation, which links body, mind and breath, has deeper psychological and spiritual implications because it stimulates subtle vital energies leading to states of higher awareness.

Larry Payne and others
Yoga for Dummies

Chapter 3

Surya Namaskar: Benefits

'The sun is revered the world over as a symbol of energy and vibrant life. One of the most popular routines in the advanced yoga teacher training, the 'Surya Namaskar' has showing gratitude to the sun as its essence. It also connects us to the solar powers within, activating the pingala nadi. The Surya Namaskar is a graceful sequence of twelve yoga postures performed as one continuous routine. This sequence of postures is designed to bring your body, mind and breath together to work in harmony'.

https://www.himalayanyogainstitute.com/multiple-benefits-surya-namaskar/

When you start practicing SN regularly, you can get the following benefits according to the quality of practice and appropriate execution. You will:

Physical level

- become more flexible

- reduce tightness in the body

- improve overall fitness

- strengthen bones

- acquire a flexible spinal cord

- reduce weight

- facilitate adequate stretching and compressing of the entire body

- tone the skin

Energy level

- have great energy

- become more active

- improve digestion

- improve circulation

- be able to do any activity well

- benefit all internal systems: digestive, excretory, circulatory, respiratory, nervous, endocrine and skeletal.

- improve lung function

- oxygenate cells and tissues of the body

- get better immunity

Mind level

- sleep better

- have better memory power

- reduce negative thoughts and feelings

- reduce fear and anxiety

- focus well

- calm the mind

- think better

Personality level, at this level

- you will be more confident

- you will be able to handle your challenges much better

- minor health challenges disappear

- you cope better with any situation

- you can understand yourself better

At the **Bliss level** you will be more joyful. Deep changes take place at all levels when SN is practiced with sincerity and when it is continued for a long time.

However, rather than thinking about the benefits, **practitioners should focus more on the quality of practice. SN knows what benefits it should give, when and to whom.**

How benefits happen

Surya Namaskar stretches, compresses and expands the organs; it fills air in the lungs and removes air from the abdomen. It bends and arches the spine. As a result, the connected organs are stimulated and they work better.

The expansion of the chest and contraction of the abdomen happens naturally, so that the respiratory and digestive systems become healthier.

When the abdomen compresses, exhalation happens well; when the chest expands naturally, inhalation happens. Deep breathing doesn't mean that only these two organs are benefited; oxygen spreads to all extremities, and all parts of the body are stimulated. Carbon dioxide is more effectively removed.

'Different evidence-based studies suggest that Surya Namaskar improves metabolic function, strengthens and makes flexible the musculoskeletal system, balances the endocrinal system, tunes the central nervous system, supports the urogenital system and boosts the working of the gastrointestinal system. Surya Namaskar practice revitalizes the body and keeps the mind calm, attentive and stress-free.

Dr. Amit Vaibhav
www.ssjournals.com

My Personal Experience of Surya Namaskar

'When the sun is shining, I can do anything; no mountain is too high, no trouble too difficult to overcome.'

Wilma Rudolph
www.telegraph.co.uk/health-fitness/mind

I am blessed indeed to practice three styles of Surya Namaskar (Krishnamacharya yoga style, Ashtanga yoga and Power yoga) and experience them well. I have also always had the opportunity to share them with others through my yoga classes. Hence, I am able to understand and feel Surya Namaskar practices better.

The moment I decide to practice SN, thoughts and feelings changes and the mind become calm. The connection with SN itself brings changes in me. Before I start, I will be in silence for a few seconds or I take a few breaths.

The first few rounds are slow; it takes time to get the feel of the practice and also to synchronize breath and movement. To bring this connection, I need to focus and this helps me to be fully in the present. Then things change, and I go with the flow accordingly.

Sometimes I stay one or a few breaths in some of the steps of SN; sometimes I bring a new asana into it; sometimes I bring sound; and sometimes, I slow down by using counts in order to increase the duration of the breath. Sometimes I close my eyes during SN practice: it gives a much better focus and is a different experience.

After SN practice, things seem new. So many changes happen in me and I am not able to put all the experiences gained through SN in words. Often, I cannot understand exactly what happened within me! But I am able to feel the positive changes and I feel far better after the practice. Can anyone comprehend and share the internal and external experiences of SN fully?

I start my practice with the Kneeling Sequence (which is the easy version of Surya Namaskar) when I am tired or feel too stiff. When I feel full of enthusiasm and am energetic, I start with the tougher version of Surya Namaskar, sometimes also introducing jumps. Whatever may be the version, soon I will be different and positive and ready to move on to other activities.

To master the jumping version of SN, it took me a few weeks. Even though I am now able to do the jumping from the beginning, initially the flow was not good and graceful. I had to practice it over and over, and it took me three months to master the jumping sequence to my satisfaction.. Now I enjoy this practice so much that when others see my jumping sequence, they go, 'Wow'!

Many yoga teachers and students do only a few rounds of SN when they do not find time for a long practice. Even after the short practice they feel good, energetic and able to execute their activities well. I have seen the joy in manywhen they do Surya Namaskar practice.

When I do Surya Namaskar in the early morning, it really makes the day very active. It gives me immense benefits, and I feel grateful for that. There are so many good things that happen to us almost all the time. I have also been seeing the changes and benefits in yoga practitioners in general and particularly in young adults, when they practice Surya Namaskar regularly.

A few specific experiences of mine:

- SN makes me more active

- I become more positive

- I become more energetic

- I become more focused after a few rounds

- I feel healthier

- It increases the length of my breathing

- I feel happy during and after practice

- I become more conscious of my activities

- I become more calm

- I am able to direct my energy better

- My whole system remains involved and nothing is left out during the practice

- I feel I do the best thing in the moment

- Every step gives me a different experience

- Every moment makes me somehow better

- When I close my eyes and do it slowly, it becomes an amazing journey and experience.

- I feel peaceful.

- I feel cleansed

- My inner chatter reduces and silence increases

- Dullness reduces and my fitness increases

- I feel motivated

- In the long run, my habits change for the better

After experiencing and knowing more about Surya Namaskar; after hearing so much from yoga practitioners and teachers; and after reading so many books and articles about it… I have also been inspired to write about my experiences. With this book I am sharing my way of approaching SN in order to reach as many people as possible.

Teaching Experience

My yoga classes are meant for fitness and general health. Hence, almost all the participants are able to do SN. However, students are of all types, and many have preferences.

For instance, since one round of SN has many steps, some may get confused in the sequence of the steps in the beginning. Such students often stop to watch others and then continue.

Some students practice SN like a dance – gracefully, in harmony with the breath. Some would like to increase intensity so that they sweat during SN; others do the sequence very slowly to increase the duration of the breath, while still others like to stay in adhomukhasvanasana. A very few people love to do SN like a cardio workout – very fast with many rounds.

 School students tend to compete with each other. So they like to do many more rounds of SN. Sometimes we may ask one student to correct another. All students enjoy correcting others and finding faults in others' practice.

Those who have learnt in other schools of yoga find this style somewhat new. They take time to adapt – to familiarize themselves. No matter which style, it will take time to coordinate breath and movement, but this will follow if practice is regular and sincere.

People who are new to yoga will find it tough in the initial stages. Experienced people expect to do more rounds of SN. Some days we choose to do only SN with pranayama – of course there will be rest in between. On these days, we start with two steps, then three steps, then four steps once or twice and then we include all the steps. Many enjoy this progression.

Sometimes people choose the kneeling sequence to practice on their own in the group classes. For example, one student who had severe back pain chose the kneeling sequence in order not to aggravate the pain.

Sometimes we may use counts in each step, so that the duration of the inhalation or exhalation is increased: we can use numbers, the OM sound or the Ah sound or other mantras to increase the duration of the breath. Using sound has many benefits, too many to list here, but importantly, it allows the student to be in the present. Their mind does not wander and they derive greater benefit from the practice

In my experience, there will most often be a change after practicing SN.

People who feel dull and weak, have a bit of pain, have less energy and so on like to do a mild practice. But after a few rounds of SN, they change their mind and want to slowly increase the intensity of the practice. Their communication is also different. Many will express their feelings, how energized they feel and how they have changed.

Those who have health issues and push too much will have discomfort, and sometimes they are not able to do SN with the group. We stop them from doing SN and suggest to them to do other suitable asanas at the moment. They can come back to SN later.

There is a website called Petheos; it says that if someone practices SN daily, systematically, correctly and faithfully and according to the instructions, it will create 34 benefits. All 34 are listed. You can check it here: https://www.patheos.com/blogs/hindu2/2015/01/sun-salutation-benefits-of-practicing-sun-salutation/

Healthy practices like Surya Namaskar is needed in today's world more than ever: not just knowing it, but also practicing Namaskar well and making it a part of our life. Many yoga practitioners and teachers feel that SN has brought a lot of difference to their lives.

Chapter 4

Guidelines

'Generally, people understand Surya Namaskar as an exercise: it strengthens your back, your muscles, etc. Yes, it definitely does do all that and more. It is quite a complete workout for the physical system – a comprehensive exercise form without any need for equipment. But above all, it is an important tool that empowers human beings to break free from the compulsive cycles and patterns of their lives.'

Sadhguru https://isha.sadhguru.org/

Before Surya Namaskar

Preparation helps us to focus and our practice becomes better.

- Preparation always helps to have better focus

- Connect with yourself by putting other things aside

- Ensure your stomach is empty

- The morning time is ideal for SN practice

- If not possible, please practice in the evening

- Start at a slow pace and ensure that every step is addressed well

- If your body is too tight, you may do warm-up exercises before SN practice.

- You may chant before starting the practice to bring your mind into the practice if you wish.

- Give a 15-minute break if you have had anything to drink.

- Take a short rest then start the practice if you are tired.

- Give a 10–to-15 min. gap to bring your system to normalcy, if you went for a walk or a jog.

After Surya Namaskar

- Take rest for a few minutes.

- Take a few deep breaths.

- Observe the impact of the practice.

- Do pranayama with guidance.

- Sit silently for some time to hold the experience.

- Watch your breath in silence for a few minutes.

Do's and Don'ts

- Have a clear idea of what you are going to do.

- Get guidance from an experienced yoga teacher.

- Start at a slow pace with fewer rounds of SN in the beginning.

- Practice it with a group of people if you so choose.

- Use the breath properly and be in the present fully.

- Now and then stop and check your practice and correct it if needed.

- If something unusual happens, stop the practice and consult a yoga teacher.

- Start writing about your SN experiences to see the changes clearly.

- Listen to your body; don't push too much initially.

- Avoid SN practice when you are not well or too tired.

- If you have health issues, consult a yoga teacher for yoga therapy.

When not to practice Surya Namaskar

- When your stomach is full

- When you have a stomach ache

- After travelling at night

- In the hot sun

- When you have a severe headache

- When you have spinal cord-related issues.

- During menstruation

If you have any of the following ailments, you should not practice SN.

- Heart disease

- Giddiness or vertigo

- High blood pressure

- Pain in the neck, shoulders and spinal cord

- Hernia

- Severe swelling of the feet

- Migraine

- Epilepsy

- Prolonged health issues

- Pregnant women should also avoid SN.

Chapter 5

Surya Namaskar Practices

'Practice of Surya Namaskar…is capable of rendering human life heavenly and blissful. By means of it, people can become joyous, experience happiness and contentment, and avoid succumbing to old age and death'.

Pattabbhi Jois, Yogamala

For beginners

- Beginners may start with six rounds of SN.

- Take rest lying on the back for 1–3 minutes

Time: 10 to 15 minutes.

After a month or two

- Practice 8 to 12 rounds of SN.

- Rest 1–3 minutes (seated or lying).

- Do deep breathing 3–5 min (seated).

- Sit in silence 2–5 minutes

Optional

- Watch the breath

- Do long exhalation

- Chant mantras

- Visualize.

Time: 15 to 20 minutes

For experienced persons, after 6 months

- ◆ Practice more than 12 rounds

- ◆ Rest

- ◆ Do pranayama

- ◆ Sit in silence / do meditative practice

Time: 20 to 30 minutes

Surya Namaskar: Practice I

When you are ready for SN practice, ensure the space is clean and prepared with a yoga mat or a spread. Wear comfortable clothes. Check your environment and make sure it is congenial for practice. This is the classical version.

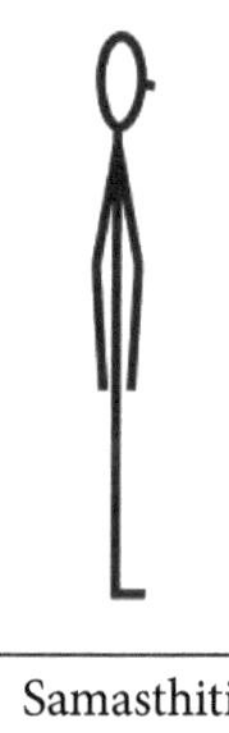

Samasthiti

Stand straight.

Feet together

Legs straight

Arms by the sides of the body

Palms facing the body

Back straight

Chin down and eyes open.

This is Samasthiti (starting position).

Take a few deep breaths in this position.

From this step go to your first movement. Start the first SN movement with inhalation.

Step-1

On Inhale: Raise the arms up from the front, hold the arms along the ears keeping the elbows straight, palms facing the front. Pause. This is raised arm position.

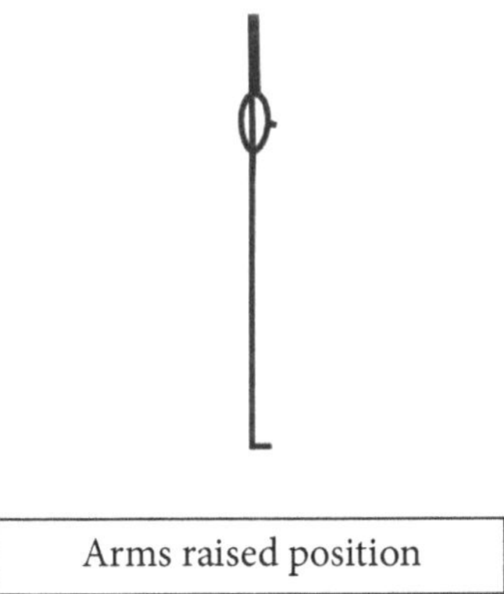

Arms raised position

Step-2

On Exhale: Bend forward and place the palms on the floor, palms by the side of the feet, touch your forehead to the knee. If you cannot, slightly bend the knee to do it comfortably. Later you may do it the classical way, with the legs straight. This is Uttanasana.

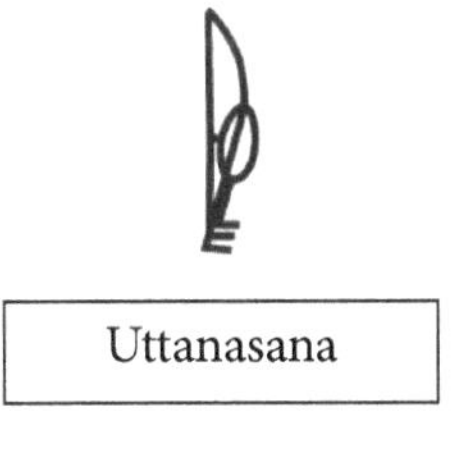

Uttanasana

Step-3

On Inhale: Stretch the left leg back, knee off the floor. The right leg is bent and the palms are on either side of the right foot. Keep the elbows straight. Look straight. Pause. This is Gotha pitham.

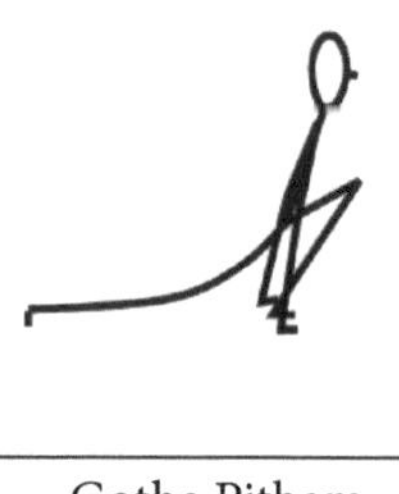

Gotha Pitham

Step-4

On Exhale: Stretch the right leg back and place it alongside the left foot and go to   Adhomukha svanasana – the downward dog position. Pause.

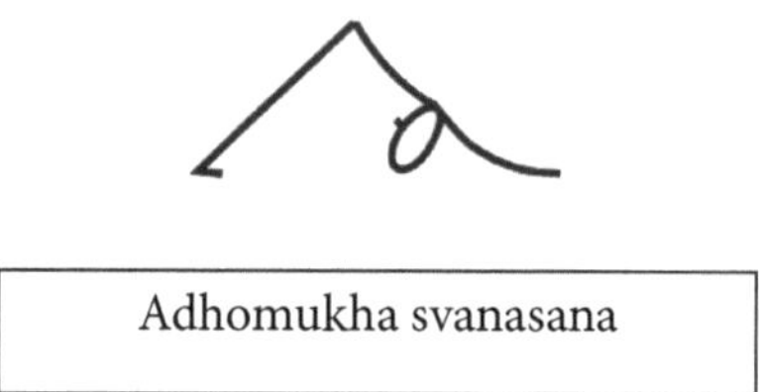

Adhomukha svanasana

Step-5

On Inhale: Bring hips down, lift head up, look straight and go to Urdhva mukha svanasana. Knees are off tte floor, feet together, knees together, arms stretched and elbows straight.

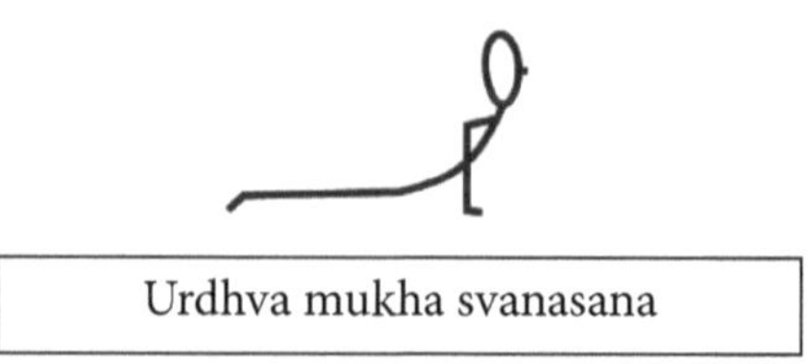

Urdhva mukha svanasana

Step-6

On Exhale: Bend forward, bring the chest and head down, place your body on the floor, stretch the arms in front of your head on the floor and join palms. This is the Namaskar position. Feel the pose by staying there a few seconds.

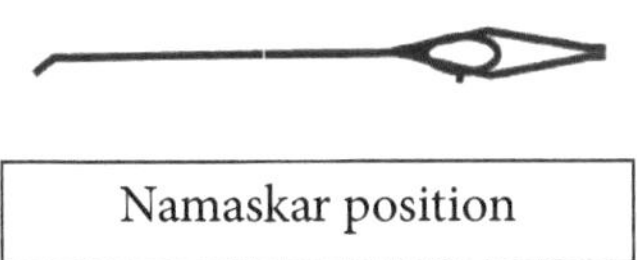

Namaskar position

We are now reversing the entire sequence to reach the starting position at the end of the next 6 steps.

Step-7

On Inhale: Bend your elbows and place palms close to the chest and lift the back and head, straighten the elbows and go to Urdhva mukha svanasana.

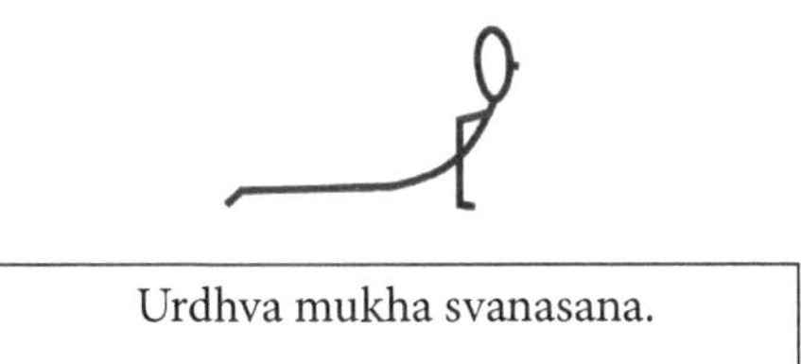

Urdhva mukha svanasana.

Step-8

On Exhale: Lift the hip and drop the head to go to Adhomukha svanasana – the downward dog position.

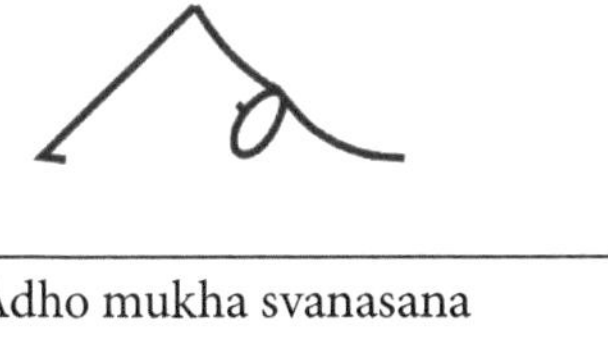

Adho mukha svanasana

Step-9

On Inhale: Bring the left leg forward and go to Godha pitham. Note that the same leg which was extended back in step 3 has to be brought forward.

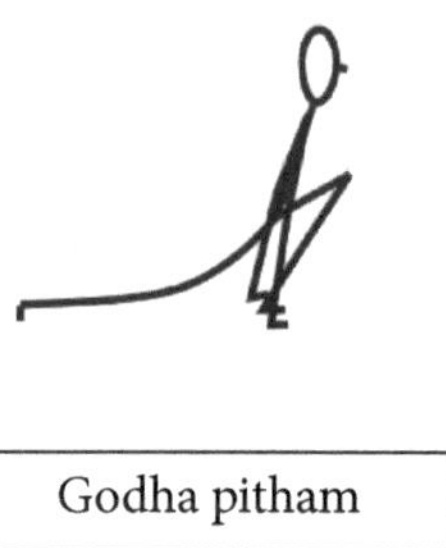

Godha pitham

Step-10

On Exhale: Bring the right leg forward and go to Uttanasana.

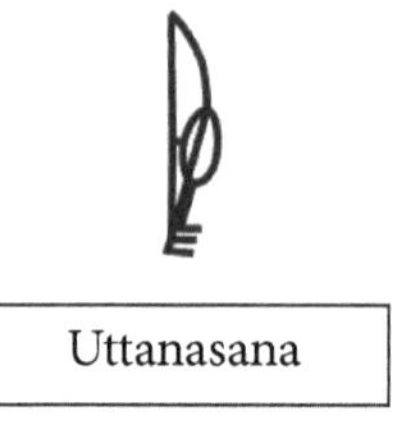

Uttanasana

Step-11

On Inhale: Arms leading the movement, slowly come up and straighten the body. Arms over the head along the ears, elbows straight and palms facing the front. Pause.

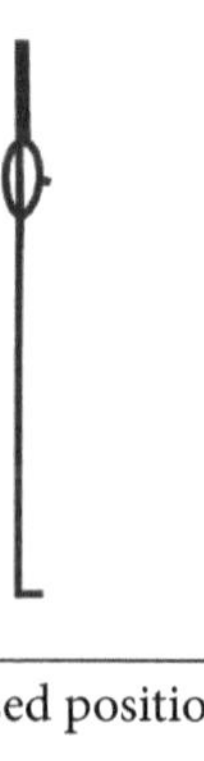

Arms raised position

Step-12

On Exhale: Bring the arms back to the sides and come back to starting point. This is Samasthiti.

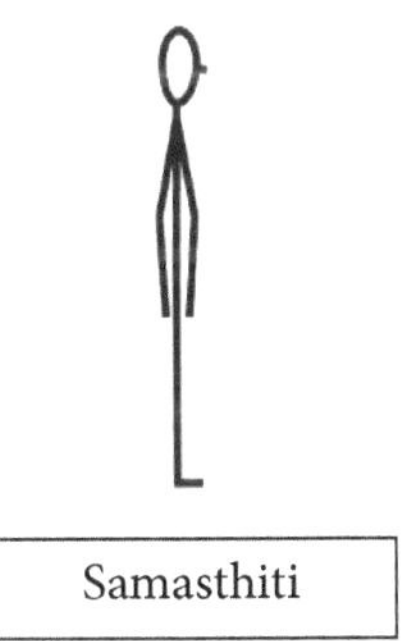

Samasthiti

Now you have done one sequence with the left leg going back. Repeat the entire sequence, now taking the right leg back in Gotha pitham. On the return, in step 10, remember to bring back the right leg back from Gotha pitham to Uttanasana. After completing both sides one round of SN is over. You may do as many rounds as you feel comfortable.

When you do SN for the first time, do it slowly to feel the steps well and co-ordinate the breath with the movement. Then once you are familiar with SN you may speed up to do more rounds and make it like a cardio workout.

If you find this practice difficult or if you feel any pain, there is a milder version of SN, which is also a very good sequence. It is very unique in the Krishnamacharya Yoga tradition.

SURYA NAMASKAR - PRACTICE 1

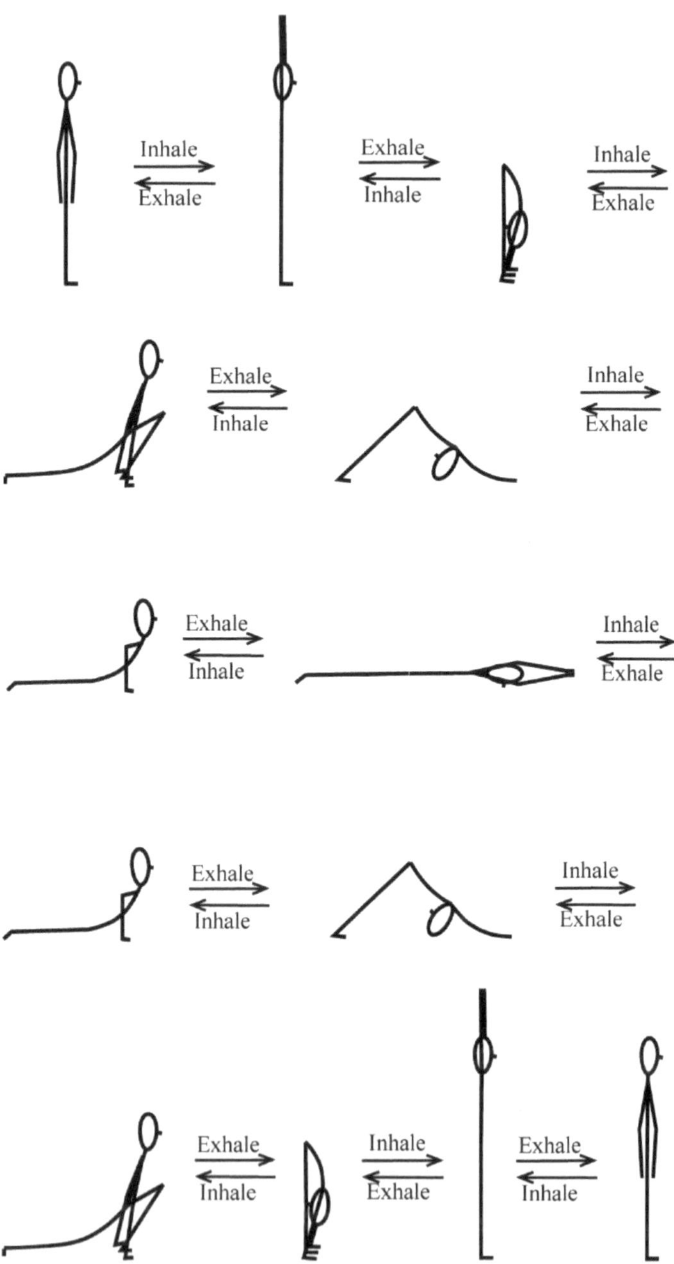

SN Practice – II

The Kneeling Sequence

Initially, if you find the classical version very difficult, you could start with this easy version. However, the goal is to do the classical practice as soon as you are able. This is very good for flexibility and one may also split it into two if you find there are too many steps.

Fold the legs and sit on the feet in Vajrasana (diamond posture). Shoulders relaxed, back straight, palms rested on the thighs, body well seated on the feet and feet together. When you are ready start the movement slowly, along with the breath.

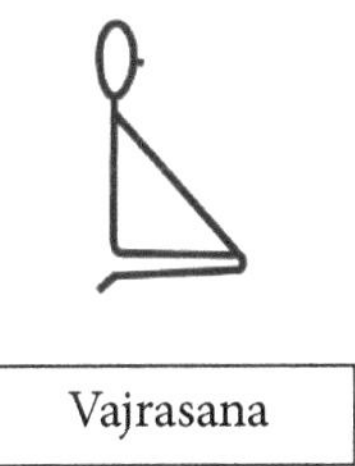

Vajrasana

Step-1

On Inhale: Rise on the knees and simultaneously raise the body, arms above the head stretched along the ears, elbows straight and palms facing the front. Feel the position pleasantly for a second or two. This is the arm raised position.

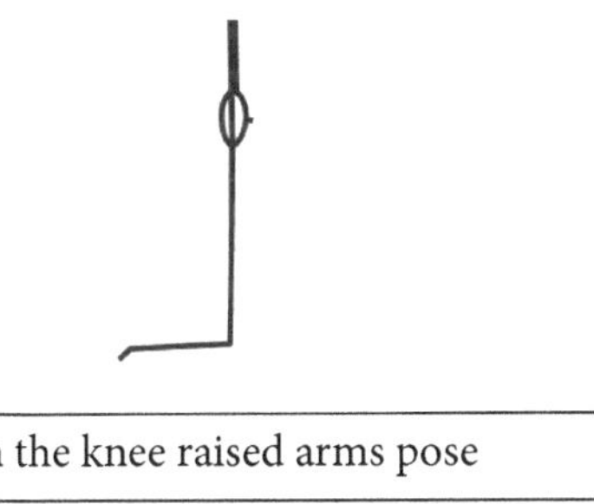

On the knee raised arms pose

Step-2

On Exhale: Bend forward and place the palms and forehead on the floor with arms stretched and back relaxed. Pause. This is Vajrasana forward bend

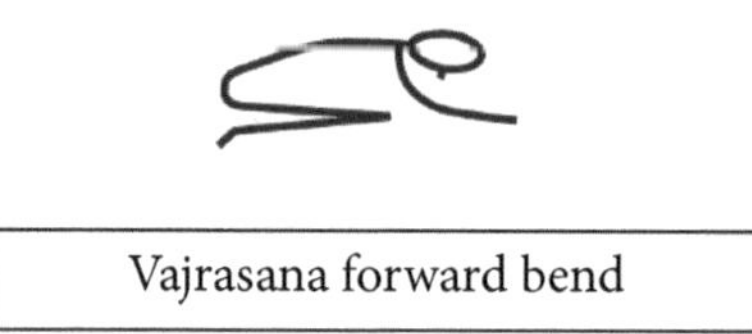

Vajrasana forward bend

Step-3

On Inhale: Raise the torso up, move forward and arch your back, legs and arms perpendicular to the floor. Palms are placed at shoulder level and the feet a little separated. Look straight. This is Cakravakasana. Then slowly and smoothly go to the next step.

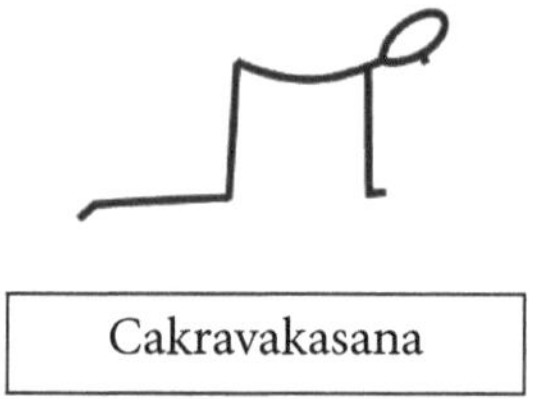

Cakravakasana

Step-4

On Exhale: Place feet firmly on the floor, lift the hips up and bring the chest and head down. Place the crown of the head on the floor if possible, arms stretched with palms on the floor. This is called Adhomukha svanasana (downward facing dog pose). Feel the pose for a second or two.

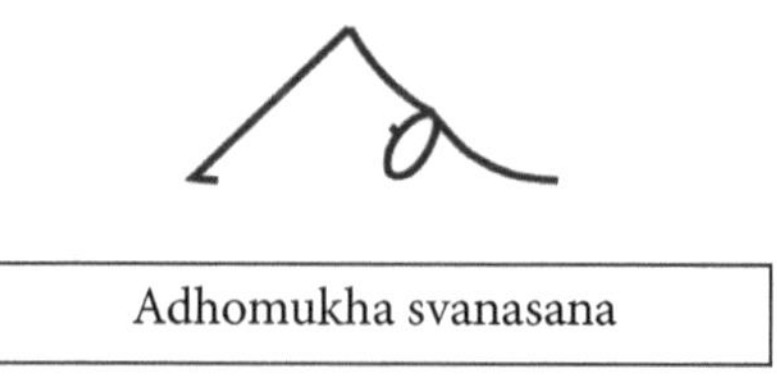

Adhomukha svanasana

Step-5

On Inhale: Lift the chest and head up and lower the hips down with arms stretched and the body balanced on the palms and toes. It is called Urdhva mukha svanasana (upward facing dog pose). Feel the step well.

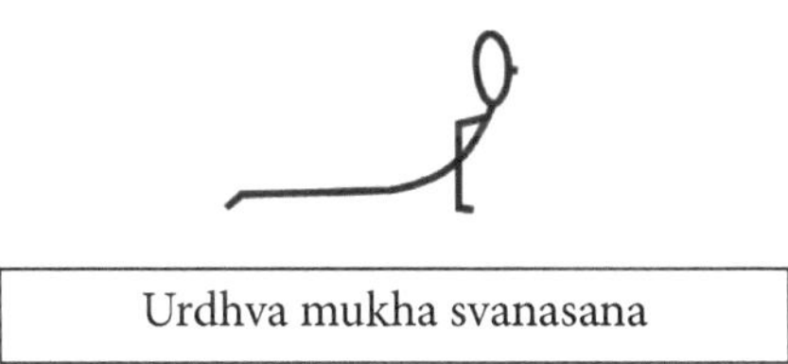

Urdhva mukha svanasana

Step-6

On Exhale: Bend forward, bring the chest and head down, place your body on the floor, stretch arms in front of your head on the floor and join palms. Now you are in Namaskar position. Pause.

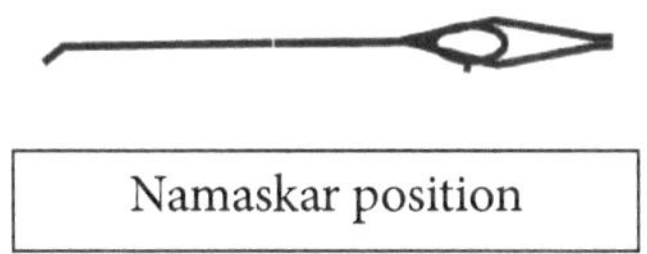

Namaskar position

We are now reversing the entire sequence to reach the starting position.

Step-7

On Inhale: Bend your elbow and place the palms close to the chest and lift the back and head, straighten the elbows and go to Urdhva mukha svanasana.

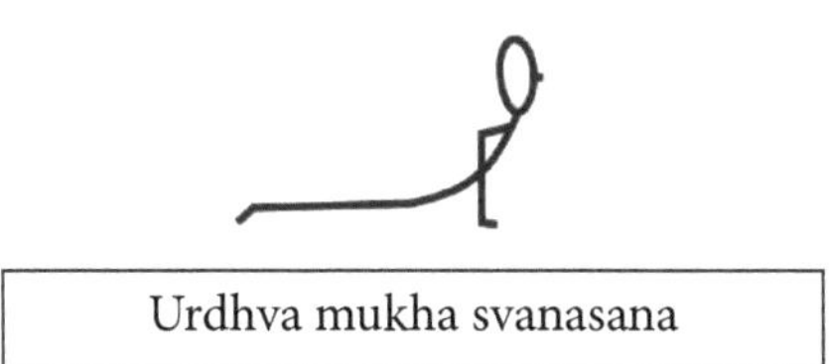

Urdhva mukha svanasana

Step-8

On Exhale: Lift the hips and drop the head to go to Adhomukha svanasana.

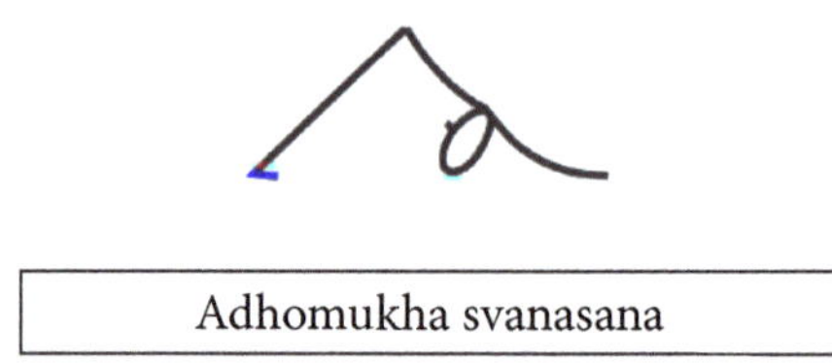

Adhomukha svanasana

Step-9

On Inhale: Drop the knees to the floor and look straight. Elbows straight. Feel the pose. This is Cakravakasana

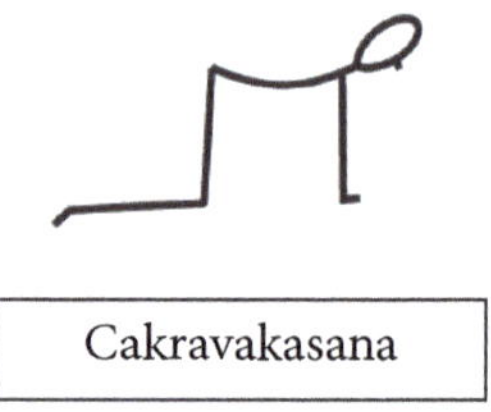

Cakravakasana

Step-10

On Exhale: Bring head to torso level and slide back to sit on the heels and place forehead on the floor between arms. This is Vajrasana forward bend.

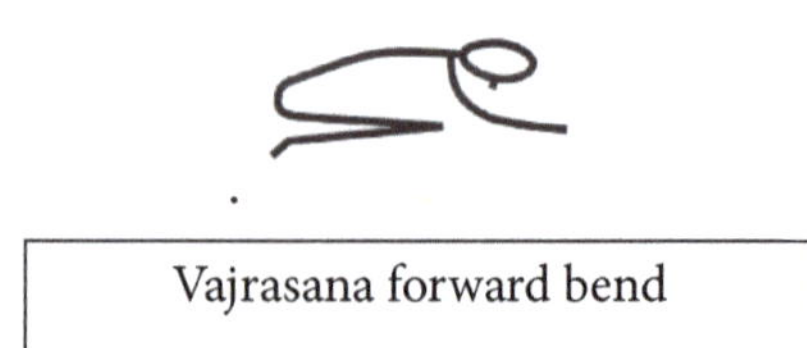

Vajrasana forward bend

Step-11

On Inhale: Slowly and steadily rise on the knees and lift the arms above the head, with the arms leading the movement. Keep the arms by the ears, elbows straight and palms facing the front. Pause.

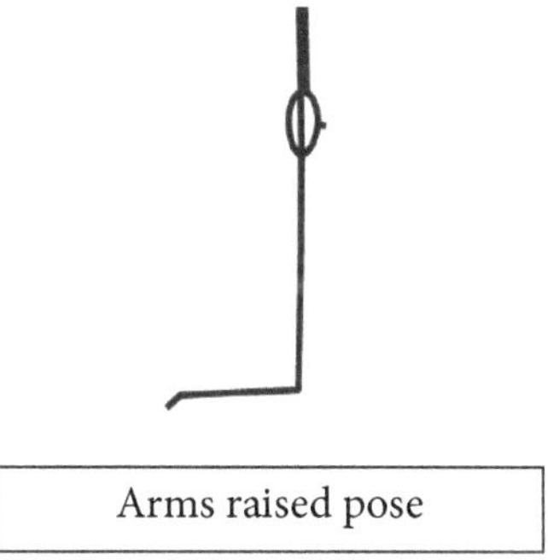

Arms raised pose

Step-12

On Exhale: Fold legs and sit on the feet, and simultaneously drop the arms back to the thighs. Keep the back straight and shoulders relaxed. Go back to Vajrasana.

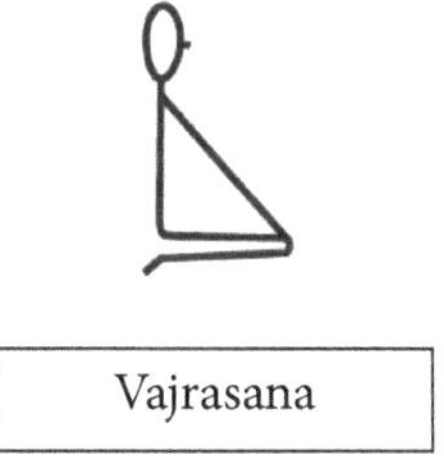

Vajrasana

This is one round of kneeling sequence of SN and you may do as many rounds as you are comfortable doing.

Complete practice - II

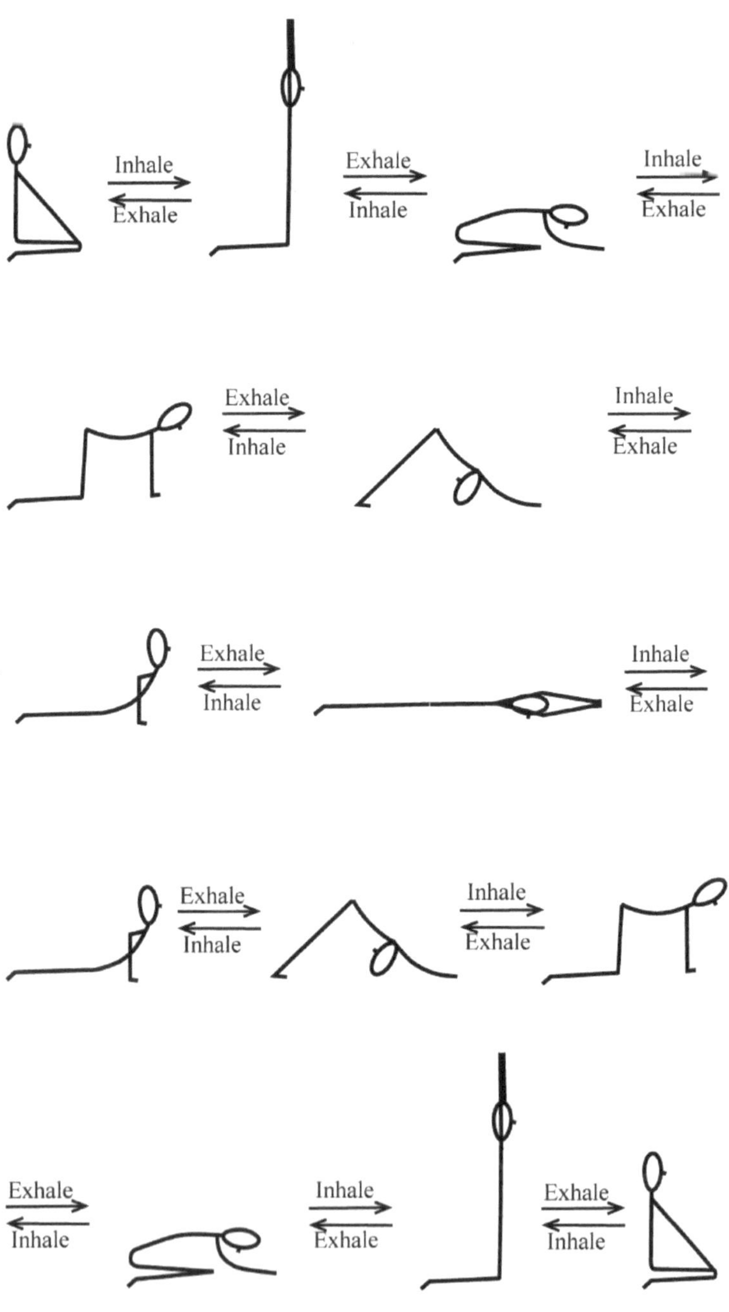

SN practice - III

Well experienced Chennai-based Ashtanga yoga teachers, Ms Srimathi and Mr Ravi, say 'only in Ashtanga yoga there are two Surya Namaskars A and B. In Ashtanga yoga practice all the practices start with this A and B. People who are fit could do these series well. It needs good health, flexibility and strength. Otherwise, they may start with the usual SN for some time and come to this later.'

In their classes, they start with these series of five rounds each of A and B. Only then do they move to other poses. As they say, the jumping is very special in Ashtanga yoga. It has to be done very smoothly, like how a cat jumps.

If anyone is able to master this style of yoga, their fitness level surely will go up, and they can do things better with that power of yoga.

Ashtanga yoga has many steps and techniques so it should be learned from an experienced yoga teacher. Here I give the simple and easy version of a jumping sequence: it is called Uttanasana Vinyasa, which has fewer steps and is similar to classical SN

Uttanasana Vinyasa (Jumping sequence)

Stand comfortably with feet together, legs straight arms by the sides of the body and eyes open – this is the starting position.

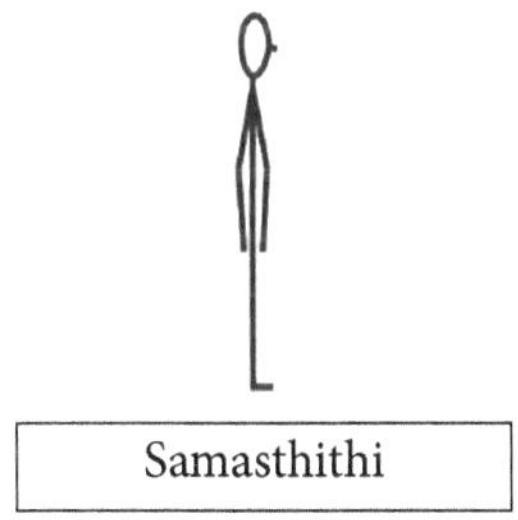

On Inhale: Raise the arms up from the front, arms along the ears, keeping the elbows straight, palms facing the front and pause.

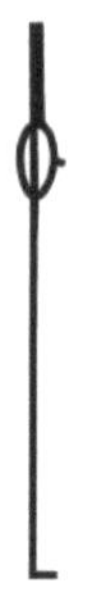

Raised arm position

On Exhale: Slowly bend forward and place the palms on the floor (palms are placed by the side of the feet). Touch the knee with the forehead. (If this is not possible, you may bend your knees slightly.)

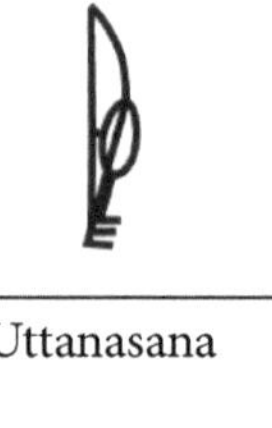

Uttanasana

From this position you are going to jump to another step. So, please be more attentive and alert.

Shift the body weight to the palms, hold the breath and jump backward with feet together into Caturanga dandasana. Place the palms on the floor under the shoulders, elbows facing up. Feet together. Place the palms and the toes firmly on the floor, and lift the body off the ground. Hold the head, neck, torso and legs straight and parallel to the floor with knees off the floor. Knee straight and off the floor.

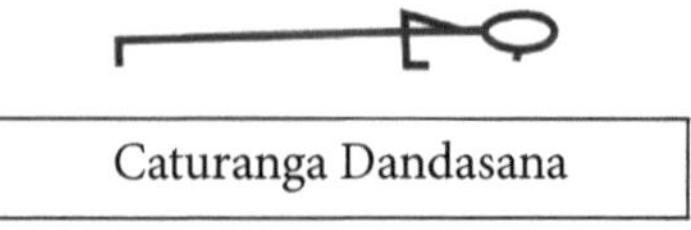

Caturanga Dandasana

On Inhale: Lift the head and back and simultaneously straighten the torso to go to Urdhva mukha svanasana (knees of the floor and elbows straight)

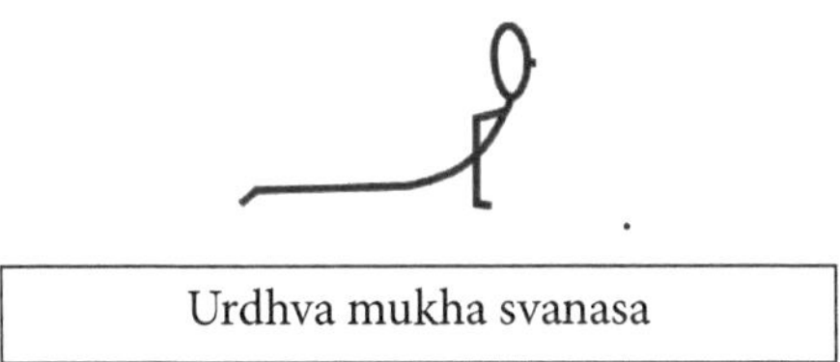

Urdhva mukha svanasa

On Exhale: Lift the hip and drop the head to the floor and go to Adhomukha svanasana

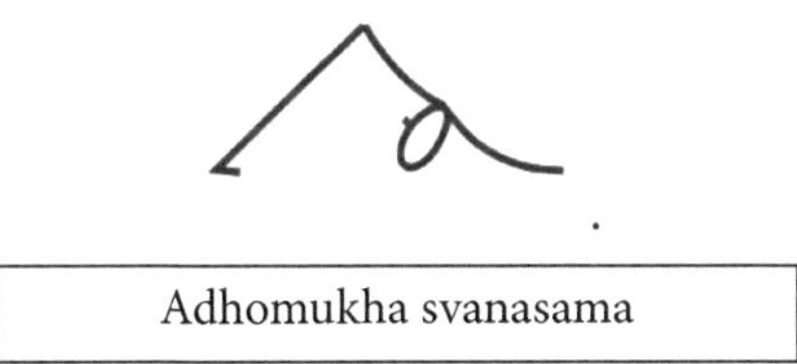

Adhomukha svanasama

Shift the body weight to the palms, hold the breath and jump forward and go to Uttanasana, the forward bent pose, or the second step.

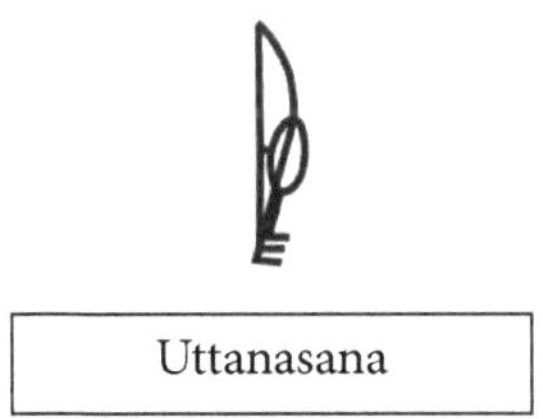

Uttanasana

On Inhale: Raise the arms over the head with the arms leading the movement and come up.

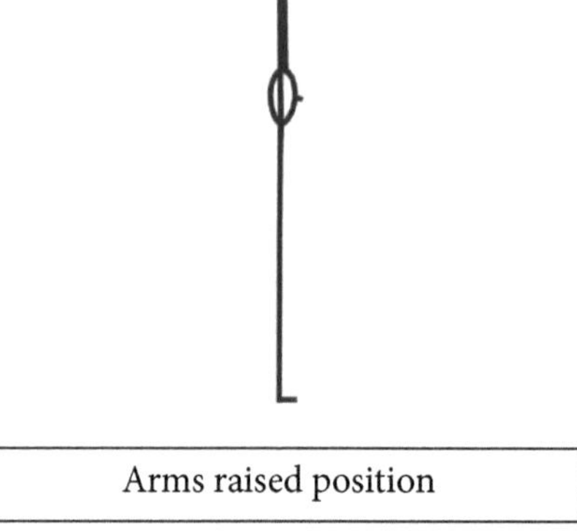

Arms raised position

On Exhale: Bring the arms back to the sides and come back to Samasthithi.

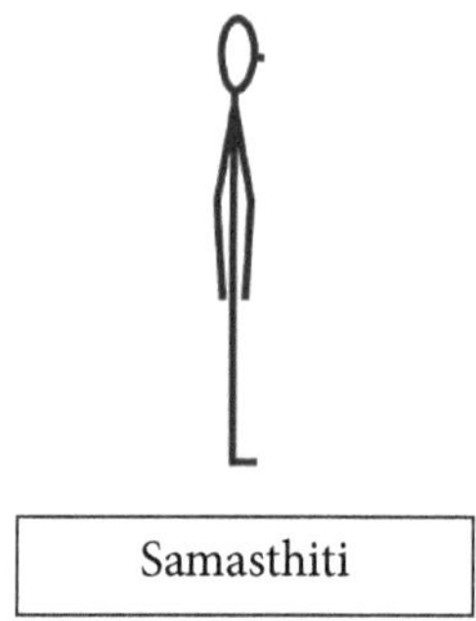

Samasthiti

This sequence has two jumps which will make you feel good. Don't do too many rounds in the initial stages. Start with a few rounds, then you may gradually increase the number of rounds especially after having mastered the steps and when the flow of breath and body is smooth.

In Ashtanga Vinyasa there are more steps that one may practice with a teacher's guidance.

Complete practice - III

<u>SURYA NAMASKAR - PRACTICE 3</u>

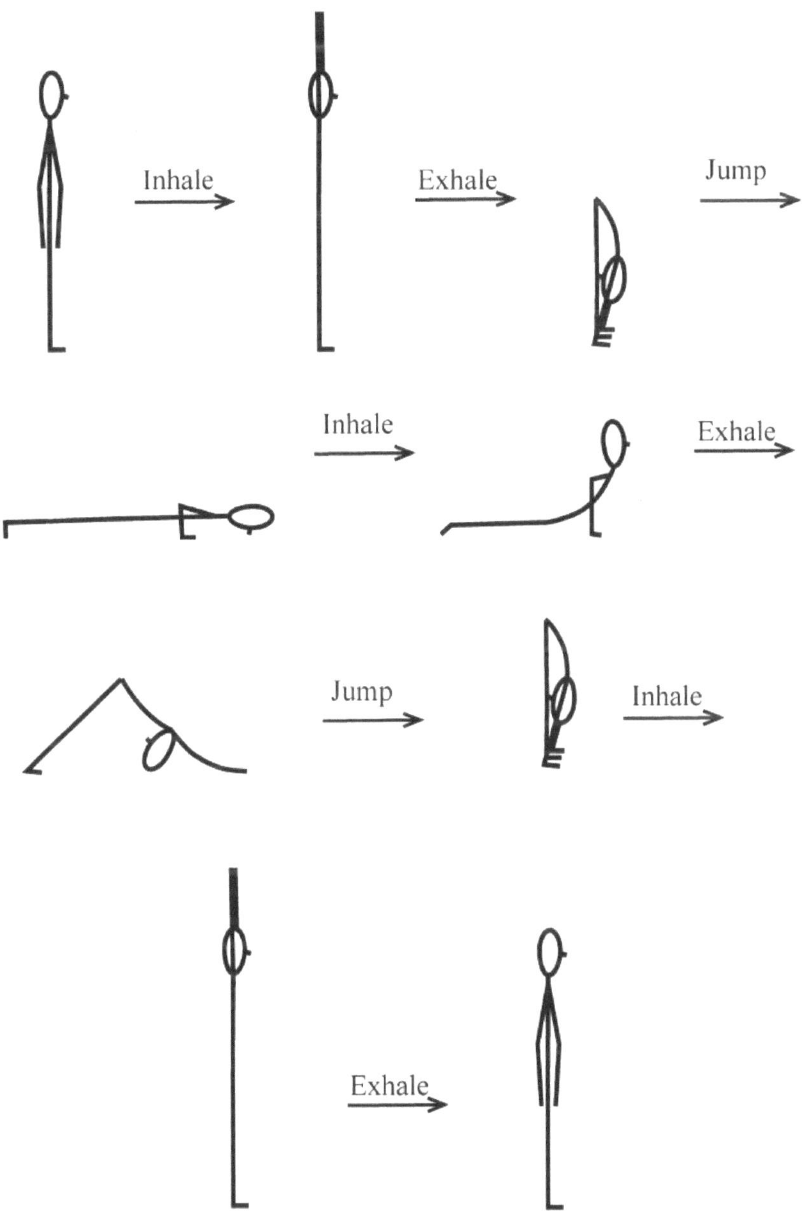

This sequence has two jumps which will make you feel good. Don't do too many rounds in the initial stages. Start with a few rounds, then you may gradually increase the number of rounds especially after having mastered the steps and when the flow of breath and body is smooth.

In Ashtanga Vinyasa there are more steps that one may practice with a teacher's guidance.

A few points to remember

Combinations

When you feel bored or like to do new ways of Surya Namaskar practice, you may practice with a combination of two or three variations.

- While doing normal SN, from Adhomukha svanasana, one may jump to Uttanasana.

- You can start the easy version of SN from Vajrasana. After a few rounds, when you feel a little more energetic, you can shift this to the classical SN by going from Adhomuhkha svanasana to Godha pitham and then Uttanasana. You can then continue in the classical method.

- You can also do the reverse, by going from Audhomukh svanasana to Chakravakasana.

- Sometimes one may start with kneeling and end with jumping.

Steps:

1. Sit in Vajrasana - Hips on the heels, toes pointing outward, palms placed on the knees

2. On Inhale : go on your knees and raise arms up

3. On Exhale: go to Vajrasana forward bend - bend forward, place arms on the floor, arms stretched, elbows straight, forehead on the floor)

4. On Inhale: go to Cakravakasana- raise torso up, move slightly forward, arch your back and look up

5. On Exhale: go to Adhomukha svanasana - lift knees off the floor, raise hips up, place feet firmly on the floor, drop head down to floor, arms stretched.

6. On Inhale: go to Urdhva mukha svanasana - bring hips down, lift chest and head up and look up straight, arms and elbows straight, knees off the floor.

7. On Exhale: Bend forward, bring the chest and head down, place your body on the floor, stretch arms in front of your head on the floor and join palms. Now you are in Namaskar position. Pause.

8. On Inhale: Go back to Urdhva mukha svanasana (Step 6)

9. On Exhale: go Adhomukha svanasana (Step 5)

10. Hold breadth and Jump to Uttanasana - shift weight to the palms and gently jump to bring feet together in between the palms. forehead touching the knees

11. On Inhale: raise arms up, come up, arms along the ears and elbows straight

12. On Exhale: go to Uttanasana - bend forward and place palms on either sides of the feet, forehead touching the knees

13. Hold breadth and Jump to Adhomukha svanasana- shift weight to the palms and gently jump back with feet together, feet placed firmly on the floor, hips raised and drop head to the floor, arms stretched (Step 5)

14. On Inhale: go to Cakravakasana- bring knees down, arch your back and look up (Step 4)

15. On Exhale: go to Forward bend Vajrasana - bend forward, place arms stretched on the floor, elbows straight, forehead on the floor (Step 3)

16. On Inhale : go on your knees and raise arms up (Step 2)

17. On Exhale: go to Vajarasana- brings arms down and sit on your heels, palms placed on the knees (Step 1)

Stay in some steps

After practising a few months and reaching reasonable flexibility, sometimes staying for a few breaths in some of the steps would be a good idea. It helps to strengthen some part of the body.

- For example, to strengthen the arms you may stay in Urdhva mukha svanasana

- to work with abdomen and hamstring stay in Adhomukha svanana

- To stretch the back muscles stay in Uttanasana.

Chapter 6

Finally, a few words

These are a few basic SN sequences. There is also Sivanada Yoga, and Bihar school of yoga Surya Namaskars. Recently Chair SN has become popular and those who are not able to do classical SN have an option to do this.

People who are really interested and ready to make the right effort will find the right practice and benefit from it.

SN practice is a long journey. People who struggle at the initial stage will find that after a month or two their practice is very different. After a year, it will become very smooth, and will flow well. When the breath increases, the SN practice changes; when the mind calms the practice is different.

You can begin with SN and then go towards more breathing exercises, pranayama and meditative practices according to your need.

You may go deeper into the sequences by doing deep breathing, by staying in the final posture for a few breaths, by closing your eyes, by using chants and so on. You can also increase the number of rounds once you become more adept to it.

However, even the basic classical SN done regularly over a long period is best for good health.

After experiencing SN well, some of you may choose to do advanced asanas; some may be interested in knowing yoga in general and the theoretical aspect in particular. Many may choose to study

Patanjali's Yogasutra where Patanjali talks about discipline within and outside.

When you choose yoga, be aware that there are many yoga traditions and schools. Each one approaches yoga differently. You have to choose the right one for you. In every school of yoga, there are many levels and you have to begin at the right level and go further from there.

Do your research before you choose.

www.ingramcontent.com/pod-product-compliance
Lightning Source LLC
Chambersburg PA
CBHW040302240726
48664CB00006B/1349